I0468503

# Clinical Problems
# in **Chinese Medicine**
## an integrative approach

Kwan Leung Chia
BChinMed (HK), RCMP (Australia and HK)

Authored and edited by Kwan Leung Chia.

Printed by CreateSpace, an Amazon Company.

**https://www.createspace.com/**

Copyright © 2016 Kwan Leung Chia

All images in this book are the property of the author, unless otherwise noted.

All rights reserved. No part of this publication may be reproduced or utilized in any form or by any means, electronic or mechanical, including photocopying, recording, or by any information storage, and retrieval system, without prior written permission from the author.

ISBN-10: 1530926009
ISBN-13: 978-1530926008

Contact (Email): insectchia@yahoo.com.hk

Related categories: medicine; alternative medicine

---

**Distributed worldwide by and available online as eBook, Kindle eBook, and paperback at:**

Amazon.com
**http://www.amazon.com/**

Amazon Europe
**http://www.amazon.co.uk/gp/gateway-eu**

CreateSpace eStore
**https://www.createspace.com/**

Clinical Problems in Chinese Medicine

# DEDICATION

This book is dedicated to my family who supported and financed me to study aboard for a medical degree after I completed my undergraduate degree in Chinese medicine.

# CONTENTS

# PREFACE

The undergraduate curriculum of Chinese medicine usually involves around 70% of traditional medicine and 30% of biomedicine. The education of biomedicine mainly focuses on basic medical sciences, for example, physiology, anatomy, pathophysiology, histology, and statistics, etc. Meanwhile, the educational component of biomedicine from a clinical perspective appears to be inadequate or inappropriate. Since I started to learn Chinese medicine, I have been having an unanswered question: how can I use the biomedical knowledge and clinical skills in my Chinese medicine practice to optimise clinical assessments and managements? What should we learn? What should we not learn? If we should learn a particular topic, to what extent should we learn?

After I obtained my undergraduate degree in Chinese medicine in Hong Kong, I was fortunate enough to be able to study a medical degree in Australia. My learning experience in the medical school provided me with insights of what level and content of biomedicine knowledge and skills are useful to Chinese medicine physicians and helpful with their clinical services.

In fact, there are several aspects in clinical biomedicine that can be useful in Chinese medicine practice. These include (1) history taking using a systematic approach, at medical graduate level; (2) physical examination skills, at junior medical officer level; (3) systematic approach to read x-rays films and indications for imaging, at junior medical officer level; and (4) commonly used medications, particularly the side-effects, which can be the chief complaint of patients who are seeking Chinese medicine service; and (5) management principle, with a focus on the non-pharmacological aspect, which can be easily integrated into your Chinese medicine management plan.

This book uses interactive clinical vignettes to illustrate how biomedicine knowledge and skills can be integrated into your Chinese medicine management plans. Because these cases are modified from real clinical encounters, Chinese medicine practitioners are likely to encounter similar patients in their daily practice. More cases and information will be added in future editions.

This book does not purport to be an exhaustive text on clinical biomedicine or Chinese medicine. Therefore, readers should not expect too much information about Chinese medicine theory, assessments, and treatments. Instead, this book will try to supplement the part that conventional Chinese medicine case vignettes do not cover.

Kwan Leung, Chia
BChinMed (HK), RCMP (Australia and HK)
Adelaide, South Australia
April 2016

# Cottony feeling in the tongue in a 50-year-old man

A 50-year-old man presents with a two month history of a cottony feeling in the tongue. This has been constant and not painful. His general practitioner (GP) prescribed a five day course of antibiotics which was not helpful with the problem. He also consulted a Chinese medicine practitioner (CMP) and has been taking herbal remedies for two weeks with minimal improvements. His appetite was poor because of the problem. He also complained fragmentation of sleep and lack of energy. No night sweat. Bowel motion once or twice per day. He is an ex-smoker. The swelling is shown in Figure 1.1.

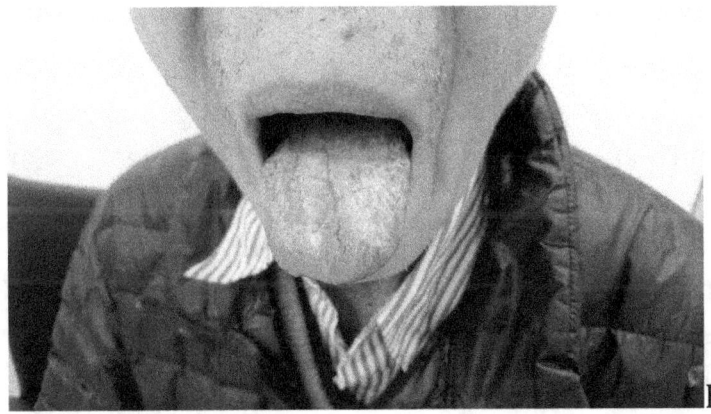

Figure 1.1

Q.1 Describe the abnormality in the photograph. What is the diagnosis?

Q.2 What further information would you like from the

history?

Q.3 What are the key features of a problem-oriented examination of a patient with suspected fungal infection?

Q.4 What is the pathophysiology in terms of biomedicine and Chinese medicine theory?

Q.5 What advise will you give the patient?

## Answers

**A.1** There is a creamy white, slightly raised lesion on the tongue. This is an oral candidiasis or oral thrush.

**A.2** You will want to know about the following:

- Any recent stressful events or cancer cachexia?
- Past medical history of any systemic illnesses, sexually-transmitted diseases and malignancies?
- Family history of malignancies or immunodeficiency?
- Medication history such as long-term steroid use, immunosuppressant, and drug abuse (sharing of needles)?
- Although asking about sexual history can be embarrassing, specific inquiry will include risky sexual behaviour and human immunodeficiency virus infection.
- Details regarding previous visits to GP and CMP.

**A.3** You will want to inspect the oral cavity, more specifically the inner cheek. Sometimes oral thrush may spread to the roof of the mouth, gums, tonsils, or the back of the throat. You will also want to examine the nails and conjunctiva to exclude anaemia, feel for the lymph nodes, and palpate the abdomen to confirm if there are any signs for systemic illnesses such as malignancies or infections. As a CMP, you should also feel the radial pulse.

**A.4** Oral candidiasis is a consequence of overgrowth of fungus Candida albicans. Candida is a normal flora in the mouth. Oral thrush can affect anyone but more likely to occur in people with suppressed or weakened immune system, such as babies, old people, and cancer patients. In Chinese medicine, external contraction of pathogenic dampness or turbid pathogen alone or combined internal dampness due to deficiency of the spleen and kidney with decreased fluid transportation and transformation and resultant water stagnation can lead to the problem in this case, and therefore, it should be treated with Chinese herbal medicine accordingly.

**A.5** Concomitant use of Chinese herbal medicine and anti-fungal can be considered, because the initial five day course of anti-fungal agents was unlikely to be adequate to eradicate the fungus. Good compliance with treatment is important, as poor compliance can lead to the lesion to spread downward into the oesophagus – Candida oesophagitis.

# Revision Points

- Oral candidiasis is a spot diagnosis. There is creamy white, slightly raised lesion on the tongue. Inner cheek and the rest of the oral cavity can be affected.
- Disorders, medications, and other factors that can cause suppressed or weakened immune system should be excluded, despite oral candidiasis can occur in normal persons.
- External and internal dampness can be the major cause of fungal infection, and therefore, should be treated accordingly.
- Good compliance with treatment is important to prevent Candida oesophagitis.

# Abdominal discomfort in a 19-year-old gentleman

A 19-year-old young man presents with abdominal discomfort. He always suffers from very bad oral ulcers and abdominal distension. His bowel motion is once per day and the stool is solid, without blood or mucus. Appetite is usual and weight has been stable. Family history is non-significant.

Q.1 What further information would you like from the history?

> His past medical history includes margarine and a recently diagnosed Crohn's disease. 12 months ago, he was admitted to the Prince of Wales Hospital in Hong Kong for assessment of a neck lump. Thyroid disorders, enlarged lymph nodes, and thyroglossal cysts were excluded. Computer tomography showed a fistula from the oesophagus. Colonoscopy with biopsy confirmed Crohn's disease. He was hospitalized for three months, with surgical repair of the fistula and administration of corticosteroids.

Q.2 What physical examination would you like to do for a patient with Crohn's disease?

There are no signs of anaemia. His abdominal examination is unremarkable.

Q.3 What is the pathophysiology in terms of Western and Chinese medicine theory?

The patient is prescribed Pinellia Decoction to Drain the Epigastrium (半夏瀉心湯) plus. He finished the course of corticosteroids and has been taking Chinese herbal medicines for four months. His abdominal discomfort and distension are relieved. Overall, his gastrointestinal conditions have been stable.

Q.4 What advise will you give the patient?

# Answers

**A.1** This patient presents with Crohn's disease, an inflammatory bowel disease, which is also an autoimmune disease. You will want to do a gastrointestinal system review and specific enquiry of symptoms and history suggestive of autoimmune disease:

- Gastrointestinal system review: appetite, nausea, vomiting, oesophageal reflux, epigastric or abdominal discomfort, abdominal pain, distension, and flatus, urine, baseline and current pattern of bowel motion and texture of stool (hard/solid/loose), with or without tenesmus, blood, and mucus.
- External manifestation: uveitis, oral ulcers, anaemia, skin lesions, arthritis, and fistula.

- General question: weight change, night sweat/fever, sleep, energy, and emotion.
- Past medical history, recent travel, and family history of autoimmune diseases: Crohn's disease, ulcerative colitis, rheumatoid arthritis, and type 1 diabetes, etc. The time of onset, last exacerbation and consequence, current medications, and last and next follow up with his endocrine doctor or general practitioner (GP) should be noted.

**A.2** Apart from feeling the radial pulse and inspecting the tongue, you will want to look for the signs related to Crohn's disease and other autoimmune diseases. It includes inspection of general appearance for malnutrition, nails and conjunctiva for malnutrition or anaemia, eyes for uveitis, palpation of abdomen for tenderness, joints and spine for arthritis, and skin for rash/lesion. Digital rectal examination and urinalysis should also be done in GP setting, but these appear to be too much for a Chinese medicine practitioner.

**A.3** Crohn's disease is a chronic autoimmune condition that leads to inflammation of the lining of the digestive system. It can affect any part of the digestive system, from the mouth to the intestines. However, it most commonly occurs in the terminal ileum. During a remission, patient can be asymptomatic or suffer from mild abdominal discomfort. During a flare-up, patient often requires inpatient treatment. The causes of Crohn's disease are combinations of potential factors, including genetics, immune system, previous infection, smoking, and environment. In Chinese medicine, gastrointestinal symptoms often relate to a problem of the spleen, stomach, and intestines. It can be caused by external heat or dampness pathogens, in combination with stress, internal heat or dampness, or deficiency of the spleen and stomach. A Chinese medicine assessment is needed and treatment should be formulated accordingly.

**A.4** Lifestyle modification is important. It includes smoking cessation, exercise, and diet modification. Certain foods can aggravate the symptoms and signs. Patient should be advised to avoid or limit dairy products, low-fat foods, spicy foods, alcohol, caffeine, and interestingly, fibre. Fibre, such as broccoli, cauliflower, nuts, seeds, corn, and popcorn can make your symptoms worse, and therefore should be limited. A combination of Chinese herbal medicine and lifestyle modification may lead to a better outcome.

## Revision Points

- Crohn's disease is an inflammatory bowel disease and an autoimmune disease.
- External manifestation of Crohn's disease includes uveitis, oral ulcers, anaemia, skin lesions, arthritis, and fistula.
- Lifestyle modification is as important as Chinese herbal medicine treatment. Fibre should be avoided.

# Deranged liver function in a 74-year-old lady

A 74-year-old retired woman presents to the emergency department of Queen Mary Hospital in Hong Kong for an accidental founding of deranged liver function during a routine blood test at a public Elderly Health Centre. She has been taking the same concentrated Chinese medicine granules continuously for 51 days for her poor sleeping quality. She does not take any other medications or health supplements.

Q.1 What further information would you like from the history?

> She has been passing tea-coloured urine and grey stool for ten days. She does not have abdominal pain, nausea and vomiting, and changes in urine. Her appetite has been usual. There is no weight change or fever. There is no recent travel history. She had not eaten any uncooked food. There is no history of hepatitis infection or carrier status.

Q.2 What Chinese herbal medicine(s) is/are likely to be the culprit from the formula that she presents to you, which is shown in Table 3.1?

| Table 3.1. Instruction: twice per day | | |
|---|---|---|
| English Name | Chinese Name | Dose |
| Qi Bao Mei Ran Dan | 七寶美髯丹 | 5g |
| Ganmai Dazao Decoction | 甘麥大棗湯 | 5g |
| Radix Codonopsis | 黨參 | 1g |
| Citrus medica L. Var. Sarcodactylis wingle | 佛手 | 2g |
| Poria cum Radix Pini | 茯神 | 2g |
| Ligustrum lucidum Ait. | 女貞子 | 1g |
| Ziziphus jujuba Mill. var. spinosa (Bunge) Hu ex H. F. Chou | 酸棗仁 | 1g |
| Albizzia julibrissin Durazz. | 合歡花 | 1g |

Q.3 What physical examination and investigation would you like to consider?

There are no signs of jaundice or anaemia, stigmata of chronic liver disease. There is no tenderness at the abdomen and no organomegaly is found. Abdominal ultrasound shows that there is no ascites and gall stones, kidneys are normal, and the common bile duct is 0.6cm. Blood has been collected for further analysis.

## Q.4 What are your managements?

The patient is admitted under the care of general medicine unit to exclude other medical conditions. Hong Kong Poison Information Centre is consulted. Her liver function improves following cessation of Chinese herbal medicine. She is discharged after medically cleared and is asked to come for monthly follow up until normalization of her liver function. Her liver function becomes normal on day 33 after stopping Chinese herbal medicine, as shown in Table 3.2. She is keen to know how to take Chinese herbal medicine in a safer manner. A Roussel Uclaf Causality Assessment Method (RUCAM) scoring system suggests that this is a probable case of drug-induced hepatotoxicity.

| Table 3.2. Serial liver function | | | | | |
|---|---|---|---|---|---|
| Item/time | Day 1 | Day 2 | Day 3 | Day 7 | Day 33 |
| ALT (8-45 U/L) | 684 | 702 | 645 | 271 | 20 |
| AST (15-37 U/L) | 331 | 368 | 289 | 82 | 23 |
| ALP (47-124 U/L) | 81 | 84 | 82 | 71 | 58 |
| GGT (≤35U/L) | 131 | 140 | 137 | 104 | 32 |
| Albumin (39-50 g/L) | 38 | 40 | 41 | 37 | 41 |
| Total bilirubin (4-23 | 13 | 17 | 13 | 8 | 5 |

| umol/L) | | | | | |
|---|---|---|---|---|---|

# Answers

**A.1** You will want to know about the following:

- Symptoms and signs suggestive of jaundice, such as fatigue, tea-coloured urine, grey stool, abdominal pain, nausea and vomiting, and jaundice.
- Medications that can lead to deranged liver function, such as statins, intravenous drug use, and some Chinese herbal medicines.
- Past medical history, family history, drug allergy, and travel history.

**A.2** Two components in the formula are the possible causes of the deranged liver function: Qi Bao Mei Ran Dan (七寶美髯丹), which contains Polugonum multiflorum (何首烏), and Psoralea corylifolia (補骨脂). Polugonum multiflorum is well known to be hepatotoxic. Although processing can reduce its toxicity, long-term or prolonged use of it is not recommended. In 2015, a systematic review involving 450 patients summarised that 63% of patients started to have deranged liver function after taking Polugonum multiflorum continuously for ten to 60 days. Seven patients died and two patients required liver transplant surgery. Genetic defect in liver enzymes is also a possible factor, because case series had showed Polugonum multiflorum-associated hepatotoxicity in a family. Psoralea corylifolia contains psoralen and isopsoralen which are known to be hepatotoxic, particularly when it is used in a very large dose. It can also cause photosensitivity in some people. However, this herbal medicine is safe to use, as there are only few reported toxicity cases so far despite it is a very popular medicine in the community.

**A.3** Physical examination and investigations should aim to exclude medical and surgical causes of deranged liver function, and to differentiate whether the liver dysfunction is hepatic pattern, cholesteric pattern, or mixed pattern. To do that, you will do the following examination and investigations:

- Signs of anaemia and jaundice
- Stigmata of chronic liver disease
- Serial liver function test
- Coagulation profile
- Hepatitis serology
- Autoimmune assay, such as anti-nuclear antibodies and anti-smith antibodies
- Ultrasound to assess common bile duct, gall bladder, and kidneys

**A.4** You should admit the patient to the general medical ward and ask the patient to stop taking the Chinese herbal medicine. The sample of the Chinese herbal medicine and the prescription, if any, should be collected for analysis. You can also contact Hong Kong Poison Information Centre for specialist consultation if required. They will try to respond to all inquiry made by medical staff, including international calls. Serial liver function test is important and close monitoring on the ward is required, as patient's condition can deteriorate or improve during the stay in hospital. Patient can be discharged once his/her condition becomes stable and the liver function starts to improve, with regular follow up at specialist clinic until the liver function normalises.

After the liver function normalised, you can assess the causality by using RUCAM. This is an extensive scoring system used to rate the level of relationship between a medicine and hepatotoxicity. Based on the final score, the suspected drug-induced hepatotoxicity can be classified as:

- ≤0: relationship with the drug excluded
- 1-2: unlikely
- 3-5: possible
- 6-8: probable
- > 8: highly probable

Figure 3.1 showed the RUCAM checklist.

**RUCAM Causality Assessment**

Drug: _____  Initial ALT: _____  Initial Alk P: _____  R ratio = [ALT/ULN] ÷ [Alk P/ULN] = _____ ÷ _____ = _____

The R ratio determines whether the injury is hepatocellular (R > 5.0), cholestatic (R < 2.0), or mixed (R = 2.0 – 5.0)

| | | Hepatocellular Type | | Cholestatic or Mixed Type | | Assessment |
|---|---|---|---|---|---|---|
| **1. Time to onset** | | Initial Treatment | Subsequent Treatment | Initial Treatment | Subsequent Treatment | Score (check one only) |
| o | From the beginning of the drug: | | | | | |
| | • Suggestive | 5 – 90 days | 1 – 15 days | 5 – 90 days | 1 – 90 days | ☐ +2 |
| | • Compatible | < 5 or > 90 days | > 15 days | < 5 or > 90 days | > 90 days | ☐ +1 |
| o | From cessation of the drug: | | | | | |
| | • Compatible | ≤ 15 days | ≤ 15 days | ≤ 30 days | ≤ 30 days | ☐ +1 |

Note: If reaction begins before starting the medication or >15 days after stopping (hepatocellular), or >30 days after stopping (cholestatic), the injury should be considered unrelated and the RUCAM cannot be calculated.

| **2. Course** | | Change in ALT between peak value and ULN | Change in Alk P (or total bilirubin) between peak value and ULN | Score (check one only) |
|---|---|---|---|---|
| After stopping the drug: | | | | |
| | • Highly suggestive | Decrease ≥ 50% within 8 days | Not applicable | ☐ +3 |
| | • Suggestive | Decrease ≥ 50% within 30 days | Decrease ≥ 50% within 180 days | ☐ +2 |
| | • Compatible | Not applicable | Decrease < 50% within 180 days | ☐ +1 |
| | • Inconclusive | No information or decrease ≥ 50% after 30 days | Persistence or increase or no information | ☐ 0 |
| | • Against the role of the drug | Decrease < 50% after 30 days OR Recurrent increase | Not applicable | ☐ -2 |
| o | If the drug is continued: | | | |
| | • Inconclusive | All situations | All situations | ☐ 0 |

| **3. Risk Factors:** | | Ethanol | Ethanol or Pregnancy (either) | Score (check one for each) |
|---|---|---|---|---|
| o | Alcohol or Pregnancy | Presence | Presence | ☐ +1 |
| | | Absence | Absence | ☐ 0 |
| o | Age | Age of the patient ≥ 55 years | Age of the patient ≥ 55 years | ☐ +1 |
| | | Age of the patient < 55 years | Age of the patient < 55 years | ☐ 0 |

| **4. Concomitant drug(s):** | Score (check one only) |
|---|---|
| o None or no information or concomitant drug with incompatible time to onset | ☐ 0 |
| o Concomitant drug with suggestive or compatible time to onset | ☐ -1 |
| o Concomitant drug known to be hepatotoxic with a suggestive time to onset | ☐ -2 |
| o Concomitant drug with clear evidence for its role (positive rechallenge or clear link to injury and typical signature) | ☐ -3 |

| **5. Exclusion of other causes of liver injury:** | | Score (check one only) |
|---|---|---|
| **Group I (6 causes):** | o All causes in Group I and II ruled out | ☐ +2 |
| o Acute viral hepatitis due to HAV (IgM anti-HAV), or | | |
| o HBV (HBsAg and/or IgM anti-HBc), or | o The 6 causes of Group I ruled out | ☐ +1 |
| o HCV (anti HCV and/or HCV RNA with appropriate clinical history) | | |
| o Biliary obstruction (By imaging) | o Five or 4 causes of Group I ruled out | ☐ 0 |
| o Alcoholism (History of excessive intake and AST/ALT ≥ 2) | | |
| o Recent history of hypotension, shock or ischemia (within 2 weeks of onset) | o Less than 4 causes of Group I ruled out | ☐ -2 |
| **Group II (2 categories of causes):** | | |
| o Complications of underlying disease(s) such as autoimmune hepatitis, sepsis, chronic hepatitis B or C, primary biliary cirrhosis or sclerosing cholangitis; or | o Non drug cause highly probable | ☐ -3 |
| o Clinical features or serologic and virologic tests indicating acute CMV, EBV, or HSV. | | |

| **6. Previous information on hepatotoxicity of the drug:** | Score (check one only) |
|---|---|
| o Reaction labeled in the product characteristics | ☐ +2 |
| o Reaction published but unlabeled | ☐ +1 |
| o Reaction unknown | ☐ 0 |

| **7. Response to readministration:** | | | Score (check one only) |
|---|---|---|---|
| o Positive | Doubling of ALT with drug alone | Doubling of Alk P (or bilirubin) with drug alone | ☐ +3 |
| o Compatible | Doubling of the ALT with the suspect drug combined with another drug which had been given at the time of onset of the initial injury | Doubling of the Alk P (or bilirubin) with the suspect drug combined with another drug which had been given at the time of onset of the initial injury | ☐ +1 |
| o Negative | Increase of ALT but less than ULN with drug alone | Increase of Alk P (or bilirubin) but less than ULN with drug alone | ☐ -2 |
| o Not done or not interpretable | Other situations | Other situations | ☐ 0 |
| | | **TOTAL (add the checked figures)** | |

Abbreviations used: ALT, alanine aminotransferase; Alk P, alkaline phosphatase; ULN, upper limit of the normal range of values
Modified from: Danan G and Benichou C. J Clin Epidemiol 1993; 46: 1323-30.

Figure 3.1. (This form is obtained from livertox.nih.gov. This website provides detailed free information and forms about drug-induced liver injury)

## Revision Points

- Chinese herbal medicine associated poisoning is common.
- Diagnosis of herb-induced hepatotoxicity is difficult. It is a diagnosis of exclusion.
- Upon request, Hong Kong Poison Information Centre can offer useful advise to clinicians regarding diagnosis and managements.

# Abnormal menstrual period in a 41-year-old woman

Today is 23rd March 2016. A 41–year-old woman presents with menstrual period that starts seven days earlier than 'normal period'. She experiences mild menstrual symptoms, including breast swelling, emotional fluctuation, and oral ulcer. These symptoms occur before every menstruation. She is G2P1, with one miscarriage and a normal vaginal delivery of a preterm baby in 34 weeks of gestation. She is otherwise healthy and has a normal body habitus.

Q.1 What further information would you like from the history?

Her last menstrual period was 26th February 2016. Her period is usually 'seven days earlier than normal period'. Her period is regular. She has never used any hormonal contraceptive methods. She had two protected sexual intercourse by condom in the current period. Unfortunately, she did not have a menstruation diary. The menstrual blood was dark, small in volume, without blood clot, and the period only lasted for two days. She started to experience menstruation at the age of 13.

Q.2 What further details would you want to clarify?

On further questioning, the patient cannot clarify what is a 'normal period'. Despite you specifically ask several times'what is the length of your period from the first day of bleeding to the first day of bleeding of the next month?', she continues to give you the same frustrating answer. You start to use the calendar, and ask for her second last menstrual period. You finally come to a conclusion that the length of her menstrual period is around 21 days.

Q.3 What is your diagnosis?

Q.4 You continue your Chinese medicine assessment and prescribe Chinese herbal medicine for her. In addition to herbal remedies, what is your advise?

# Answers

**A.1** The key question in gynaecology is to estimate whether a menstrual period is reasonable. This can be done with the aid of a mnemonic of 'five fingers and a pencil'.

- Five fingers
  - ○ When was the first day (not the last day) of the last menstrual period?

- o   Was the last period as usual, i.e. similar to other periods in all respects?
- o   Are periods regular?
- o   If regular, what is the interval from day one of one period to day one of the next?
- o   What form of contraception was used recently and until when?
- Pencil – was the date recorded in a diary or on a calendar?

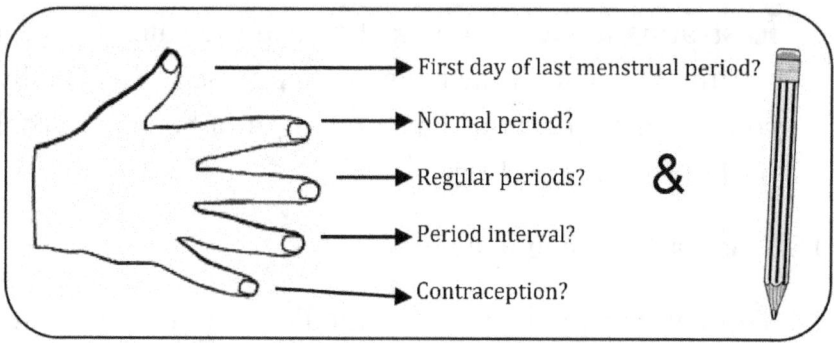

First day of last menstrual period?
Normal period?
Regular periods?       &
Period interval?
Contraception?

Other questions include the details about the menstrual symptoms, menstrual blood, pregnancy history and past medical history. You will want to know whether this occurs since the first menstrual period or after delivery.

**A.2** It is highly common to see a female patient confused with 'normal period'. You need to be patient enough to clarify the concept of 'normal period', whether it means 'normal period of the general population, i.e. 28 days', 'normal period of her usual length of period', or 'normal period from the LAST day of bleeding to the FIRST day of bleeding of the next'. Calendar is often helpful in this case.

**A.3** The diagnosis in this case is normal menstrual period.

**A.4** On top of prescribing Chinese herbal medicine for her general health, you will want to educate the patient about the concept of 'normal period' and reassure that her menstrual period is normal. Chinese herbal medicine is not going to 'delay' her menstrual period from 21 days to 28 days, as it is not possible and unnecessary. If education is not properly done, the patient would probably have consulted another practitioner next month, because of her period being the same as before.

## Revision Points

Five fingers and Pencil (calendar)
- When was the first day (not the last day) of the last menstrual period?
- Was the last period as usual, i.e. similar to other periods in all respects?
- Are periods regular?
- If regular, what is the interval from day one of one period to day one of the next?
- What form of contraception was used recently and until when?

# Generalised weakness in a nine-year-old boy

A nine-year-old boy, brought in by mother, presents with generalised muscle weakness for six months. His symptom has started for six months, following a school camp, in which he described 'being asked to do too much intense exercise'. His generalised weakness sometimes come with aching, associated with intermittent chest discomfort and nausea. He is tired despite his sleeping hour has increased. There is no recent change in weight. Bowel motion is once per day with solid stool and his urine pattern has been normal.

Q.1 What further information would you like to ask?

This boy was born as a term baby, with normal vaginal delivery. The pregnancy process was uneventful. He is the only child in the family. There are no developmental concerns. His vaccination is up to date. He is previously healthy, without history of thyroid disorder, diabetes, or neurological problems. There are no recent illness and travel. His family history includes a grandmother with thyroid disorder.

Q.2 On top of feeling the radial pulse and inspecting the tongue, what further physical examination would you like to do?

On physical examination, he is obviously overweight and appears to be tired. His speech is monotonous, with slow rate and small volume. His muscle power is five/five in all limbs. His radial pulse is regular, around 72 bpm. He has normal hair pattern, with normal texture of hair. He does not have exophthalmos, lid lag or lid retraction. There is no skin change.

Q.3 Apart from prescribing Chinese herbal medicine and acupuncture, what other managements or advises would you want to do?

A referral letter to public general outpatient department (GOPD) is written. On follow up the next week, you decided to formulate a new prescription, because the previous Chinese herbal medicine formula was not helpful with the symptoms. Meanwhile, the patient presented to GOPD and was found to have hypothyroidism.

## Answers

**A.1** A systematic approach to general paediatrics problem is often helpful to guide clinicians to reach a clinical diagnosis. In paediatrics, there is an addition of several key questions on top of the routine questions that you always want to ask an adult:

- Pregnancy: any maternal or foetal health problem during the process of pregnancy.
- Delivery: term/preterm baby, normal/complicated delivery, vaginal/C-section, and place of birth.
- Development: normal/delayed gross motor, fine motor, speech, and social developments.
- Vaccination: up-to-date vaccination, and the time of the last dose.
- Family history: health problems of the patient's sibling and parents.
- Past medical history: medical/surgical problems in infancy and childhood. You will want to specifically ask for endocrine disorders, e.g. diabetes and thyroid disorder.

**A.2** You will want to specifically perform physical examination to look for endocrine problems, mainly thyroid disorders and diabetes.

For hyperthyroidism, you will want to look for:

- General appearance: nervous/anxious, signs of recent weight loss, oily hair and skin, sweatiness, or alopecia.
- Peripheral signs: hand tremor, onycholysis, or sweaty palms.
- Radial pulse: tachycardia or irregularly irregular pulse.
- Muscle power: proximal myopathy.
- Eye signs: double vision, lid retraction, lid lag, or exophthalmos.

- Thyroid: observe the neck when patient is drinking water, and feel the thyroid from the front and behind.
- Palpitation: thyroid gland, cervical lymph node, feel the thyroid when the patient poke out tongue, and trachea.
- Percussion: percusses chest to check for lower extent of a thyroid swelling.
- Pemberton's sign: gets patient to lift both arms above head and observe for signs and cyanosis.
- Heart: auscultation listening for systolic murmur and thyroid for a bruit.
- Legs: pretibial myxoedema.
- Reflexes: hyperreflexia.

For hypothyroidism, you will want to look for:

- General appearance: slow affect, slow speech, signs of weight gain, or thick and coarse hair.
- Peripheral signs: peripheral cyanosis, swelling of skin, cool and dry skin, or pallor in palmar creases.
- Radial pulse: bradycardia.
- Carpal tunnel: Tinel's or Phalen's signs.
- Face: hypercarotaemia of skin, or thickened skin.
- Eye signs: periorbitial oedema, loss of outer third of the eyebrow, or xanthelasma.
- Tongue: enlarged tongue.
- Thyroid: observe the neck when patient is drinking water, and feel the thyroid from the front and behind.

- Palpitation: thyroid gland, cervical lymph node, feel the thyroid when the patient poke out tongue, and trachea.
- Percussion: percusses chest to check for lower extent of a thyroid swelling.
- Pemberton's sign: gets patient to lift both arms above head and observe for signs and cyanosis.
- Heart: auscultation listening for pericardial effusion and thyroid for a bruit.
- Lungs: auscultation listening for pleural effusion.
- Legs: non-pitting oedema.
- Reflexes: hyporeflexia.

For diabetes, you will want to look for:

- General appearance: signs of dehydration, i.e. sunken orbits, dry mucous membranes, and tissue turgor, moon face, pigmentation (bronzed), respiration (Kussmaul's respiration), and skin changes (acanthosis nigracans).
- Vital signs: postural hypotension, tachycardia, and hyperventilation.
- Eyes: visual acuity, cranial nerve III, IV, and VI.
- Mouth: candida infection.
- Abdomen: hepatomegaly and insulin injection sites, i.e. fat atrophy/fat hypertrophy.
- Lower limbs: hairless and atrophied skin, ulcers, skin infection, necrobiosa lipoidica diabeticorum (very rare indeed), and lower limb neurological examination for peripheral neuropathy, such as vibration sense.
- Vascular: pulses, temperature, and capillary return.

- Urinalysis and fundal examination: not done by Chinese medicine practitioner (CMP).

**A.3** Endocrine problems can be asymptomatic and if symptomatic, commonly present as highly non-specific symptoms and signs. Therefore, western medical practitioners often rely on thyroid function test, and both positive and negative result will be clinically meaningful. In Chinese medicine practice, practitioners should always maintain a high vigilance about endocrine problems. If there is any suspicion, a referral letter should be offered to western medical counterparts.

## Revision Points

- There is a number of questions designed for paediatric population and they should be asked during the consultation.
- Endocrine problems often present as non-specific symptoms and signs.
- Apart from feeling the radial pulse and inspecting the tongue, CMP can do more by performing physical examinations to look for signs related to endocrine problems.
- Apart from Chinese medicine treatments, CMP should also make appropriate and timely referral to western medical practitioners.

# Breathlessness in a 62-year-old man

A 62-year-old man presents to your Chinese medicine practice with constant shortness of breath over the last year. He also has palpitation and fatigue. He sleeps on one pillow at night. There is no dizziness, chest pain, and ankle swelling. Bowel motion is 'unstable'. He has nocturia three to four times per night. His past medical history includes atrial fibrillation and mitral regurgitation. He has poor compliance with his medication, and only takes Frusemide and Spironolactone. He does not consider valve replacement surgery and has refused to discuss it with his cardiologist. He wants you to use Chinese herbal medicine to fix his problem, because Chinese herbal medicine is said to be able to treat the 'root' of the disease.

Q.1 What further detailed information from the history would you want to know?

In terms of his activity of daily living (ADL), despite he can go to washroom on his own, he cannot go to market or walk up stair. He told you that he does not want to take too much medication and receive the surgery, because he thinks that taking too much medication is bad and open chest surgery will be dangerous. He is not on warfarin.

Q.2 What physical signs do you want to look for? What radial pulse do you expect?

He was breathless and was not able to speak in full sentence in the beginning. Now, he can talk in full sentence. He has an irregularly irregular radial pulse. His jugular venous pressure is not elevated, and the nails and conjunctiva are not pale. There is no finger clubbing or central cyanosis. Heart sounds are dual, with a systolic murmur best heard at mitral area, grade 3, radiating to aortic and axillary regions. There are no heave and thrill. Chest is clear. There are no sacral and ankle oedema.

Q.3 What advise will you give him?

Apart from prescribing a formula, you make good use of this chance to test his knowledge about mitral regurgitation (MR) and atrial fibrillation (AF). You recognise he knows nothing about his prognosis, his responsibility, and pros and cons of the surgery. After the consultation, he knows that while Chinese herbal medicine may be able to improve the quality of life, good compliance with medication is critical to improve prognosis. In addition, he understands that surgery, not Chinese herbal medicine, can treat the 'root' of the problem in this case. He will seriously consider valve replacement surgery and discuss it with his cardiologist on next follow up. He is very happy after this consultation, as he has received unexpected yet comprehensive, useful, and timely advises.

## Answers

**A.1** In this case, you will want to know the reason of shortness of breath by asking cardiopulmonary system review questions:

- Chest pain
- Breathlessness
- Dizziness
- Palpitation
- Ankle swelling
- Fatigue
- Cough
- Sputum
- Haemoptysis
- Wheezing

Meanwhile, you will want to know why the patient has poor compliance with medications and has not considered valve replacement surgery. You will also want to know the baseline, severity, and progression of the shortness of breath by asking his ADL before and after onset of symptoms.

**A.2** You will want to do a complete cardiopulmonary examination on the patient. You will look for the following signs, which are helpful to detect the cause of the symptoms and assess severity:

- Signs of anaemia: pale nails and conjunctiva.
- Signs of AF: irregularly irregular radial pulse.
- Signs of right ventricular failure: hepatomegaly, elevated jugular venous pressure, and bilateral peripheral pitting oedema.
- Signs of left ventricular failure: breathlessness, increased work of breathing, and fatigue.
- Signs of pulmonary oedema: breathlessness, increased work of breathing, pink bubbled sputum, wheezing, and inspiratory crackle on auscultation.
- Signs of valvular heart disease: cardiac murmur, thrill, and aortic bruit.
- Signs of cardiac hypertrophy: AF, heave (right), and deviation of apex beat (left).

**A.3** Patient education and advise are critical in this clinical encounter. The following key points should have made during the consultation:

- Education
  - AF significantly increases the risk of pulmonary embolism and ischemic stroke. Therefore, patient should take anti-coagulant as per instruction by his/her doctor to prevent these serious health consequences.
  - MR increases the backflow of blood to the lung and right heart. Without valve replacement surgery, this will lead to left ventricular hypertrophy, left heart failure, acute pulmonary oedema, cor pulmonale, AF, right heart failure, and eventually biventricular heart failure.

o Left heart failure presents with three classical symptoms: syncope, angina, and dyspnoea. Insufficient outflow of blood to systemic circulation can also affect blood supply to the intestines, leading to dysfunctional bowel motion.

- *Additional information for practitioners: dyspnoea carries the worse prognosis (mean survival of one to two years), then syncope (mean survival of three to four years), followed by angina (mean survival of five years).*

o Right heart failure presents with fluid overload, including hepatomegaly, ascites, and bilateral peripheral oedema.

o Medication is an essential component to prevent disease progression:

- *Additional information for practitioners: angiotensin converting enzyme inhibitor: the only anti-hypertensive proven to be able to improve survival by about 50% and protect kidney functions. Side-effects include dry cough and angioedema (as shown as enlarged tongue).*

- *Beta-blocker or calcium channel blocker (CCB): anti-hypertensives to be able to reduce symptoms of heart failure, improve cardiac remodelling (CCB only), and correct rhythm. Side-effect of CCB is mainly bilateral peripheral oedema.*

- ▪ *Aspirin and/or clopidogrel: anti-platelet medication to prevent pulmonary embolism, stroke, deep vein thrombosis, and myocardial infarction. The major side-effect of aspirin is the risk of peptic ulcer disease. Thus, proton pump inhibitor is often prescribed too.*
- ▪ *Frusemide and/or Spironolactone: diuretics to prevent fluid overload.*
  - ➢ Therefore, this patient is highly likely to develop biventricular heart failure, pulmonary embolism, and stroke without valve replacement surgery and good compliance with medication.
- • Advise and non-pharmacological treatment are as essential as your Chinese herbal medicine treatment in your management plan. Your management should include:
  - ➢ Pharmacological treatment:
    - ▪ Chinese herbal medicine
    - ▪ Western medication
  - ➢ Non-pharmacological treatment
    - ▪ Fluid restriction 1.5 L per day
    - ▪ Low salt and low fat diet
    - ▪ Sitting upright
    - ▪ Cessation of smoking
    - ▪ Affordable exercise
    - ▪ Acupuncture, as some practitioners may prefer
  - ➢ Advise:

- Good compliance with western medication as per instruction given by the cardiologist
- Chinese herbal medicine, vaccination and good lifestyle with exercise to prevent upper respiratory infection, as this can lead to fatal decompensated heart failure
- Consideration of and discussion with the cardiologist the pros and cons of valve replacement surgery
- Attendance on follow up

## Revision Points

- The danger of untreated AF is the high risk of pulmonary embolism, stroke, and deep venous thrombosis.
- The danger of untreated MR is the inevitable biventricular heart failure. Valve replacement surgery is the only intervention to be able to cure the problem.
- Non-pharmacological treatment and advise are as important as pharmacological interventions. These must not be dismissed and must be included in your management plan.

# A sprained ankle in a 52-year-old woman

A 52-year-old previously healthy woman presents at 1032 to the emergency department in Queen Mary Hospital in Hong Kong with sprained right ankle. Yesterday at around 1730, she accidentally had a very bad inversion injury when she got off the tram. She could hardly stand and presented herself immediately to a Chinese medicine practitioner (bone-setting) (CMP). The practitioner did not perform any manipulation and prescribed medicinal pads to cover the right lateral malleolus. The pads were not helpful with the symptoms. This morning, her right leg could hardly bear the weight and was very painful. Therefore, she decided to come to the hospital.

Q.1 What physical signs would you want to look for?

On physical examination, there is bruising around the right lateral malleolus. You recognise that there are bony tenderness along the distal six cm of the posterior edge of the fibula and tip of the lateral malleolus. Additionally, the patient cannot stand on her feet.

Q.2 What is your management plan?

You immediately ordered x-rays of both ankles for lateral and anteroposterior views. There is a closed transverse fracture of the right distal fibula, with medial displacement and impaction. There is no angulation. You decided to admit the patient into emergency medicine ward for closed reduction and plaster. The patient is discharged the day after and will attend follow up.

# Answers

**A.1** In trauma patient, the most important physical examination is to decide the severity of the injury. In patient with ankle injuries, you will want to look for the following to decide whether you think there is a fracture and want an x-ray (Ottawa Ankle Rule):

- Bone tenderness along the distal six cm of the posterior edge of the tibia or tip of the medial malleolus, or
- Bone tenderness along the distal six cm of the posterior edge of the fibula or tip of the lateral malleolus, or
- An inability to bear weight both immediately and in the emergency department for four steps.

If there is any pain in the malleolar zone with any one of the above, the patient should be arranged an x-ray because there is a risk of fracture. Unfortunately, her treating CMP was not able to recognise this in a timely manner and therefore delayed appropriate treatments.

**A.2** X-ray assessment is the most important part of the managements of this case. Since CMP cannot order any x-ray investigation, he/she should refer the patient to nearby emergency department or public general outpatient department. While you can continue with medicinal pads treatment, manipulation must be avoided (as it was correctly done in this case).

## Revision Points

- Ottawa Ankle Rule is very important in assessing patient with sprained ankle.
- Avoid manipulation when you suspect there is a fracture or very bad injury.
- Timely referral to medical clinic or emergency department is very helpful.

# Urinary incontinence in a 50-year-old woman

A 50-year-old otherwise healthy female presents with urinary incontinence following normal vaginal delivery of her daughter seven-year-ago. She passed diluted urine for about 15 to 20 times in daytime, associated with urgency and leakage. She usually drinks 1000 mls of fluid and she does not consume caffeine products. She has nocturia once per night. She has dry mouth and poor cold tolerance. Her sleeping quality, energy, appetite and abdomen are as usual. Bowel motion is usual, around once per day with normal solid stool. She had menopause at age 48.

Q.1 What further information would you like to know?

She has urgency, associated with leakage that can be triggered by coughing and sometimes laughing. There are no dysuria and blood in urine. There is no history of recent urinary tract infection. Her obstetrician told her that her pregnancy and delivery process weakened her ligaments that are responsible to hold the uterus and therefore her uterus may be pushing her urinary bladder. Physiotherapist was not referred at that time.

Q.2 What are the subtypes of urinary incontinence from a biomedicine perspective?

Q.3 What is the neurophysiology of bladder control from a biomedicine perspective?

Q.4 What physical examination would you like to do?

Abdomen is soft and non-tender. Bladder is not distended. Kidneys are not ballotable. There is no organomegaly. The perineum is not examined for vaginal or uterus prolapse. Her radial pulse is deep and weak. Her tongue is enlarged and pink with thin white coating.

Q.5 What is your management plan?

A clinical diagnosis of mixed incontinence is made. As you think the patient is suffering from kidney insufficiency, Liu Wei Di Huang Wan (六味地黃丸) plus is attempted. In order to objectively assess the treatment response, you ask the patient to do a urine diary. You also ask the patient to avoid stimulants such as caffeine products. You advise that patient to consider seeing a physiotherapist to learn pelvic floor exercise which may be helpful.

# Answers

**A.1** You will want to do know the following:

- Urinary system review: dysuria, discharge, change in frequency, change in colour, change in volume, hesitancy, urgency/leakage, and constipation. In

male, you will also ask for strength of the stream and terminal dribbling
- Past medical history: urinary tract infection, kidney stones, structural abnormalities, surgery, gynaecological disorders, and obstetrics problems, i.e. perineal tear during vaginal delivery
- The severity by asking the patient's activity of daily living

**A.2** Urinary incontinence is often divided into four subtypes:

- Urge incontinence (hyperactive bladder): urgency, small volume per urination and/or frequency
- Stress incontinence (weakened ligaments and pelvic floor muscles): triggered by laugh, cough, or other behaviours that can increase intraabdominal pressure
- Mixed incontinence (both): a mixture of the above symptoms
- Overflow incontinence (neurologic bladder): urinary retention/distended bladder with large volume urinary incontinence, as a consequence of damages in the upper motor neuron system

**A.3** The capacity of urinary bladder is about 400 mls with little increase in tension. The bladder contains many stretch receptors on its surface to signal the wall tension. When the wall tension increases, i.e. urine volume > 400 mls, autonomic nervous system reflex is activated (micturition reflex). This will give a sensation of fullness and an urge to urinate.

The micturition centre of the brain is in the brainstem (pons). However, cerebral activity can override micturition reflex unless the bladder is so full that its reflex signal overcome the cerebral activity. It is important to know the neurological pathway of bladder control as it can relate to acupuncture point selections, as shown in Figure 8.1:

- Sympathetic nervous system: T9 to T12 (to reflex the bladder)
- Parasympathetic nervous system: S2 to S4 (to contract the bladder)
- Somatic nervous system: S2 to S4 (to contract the external urethral sphincter to block the passage of urine from the contracting bladder to urethra

Figure 8.1

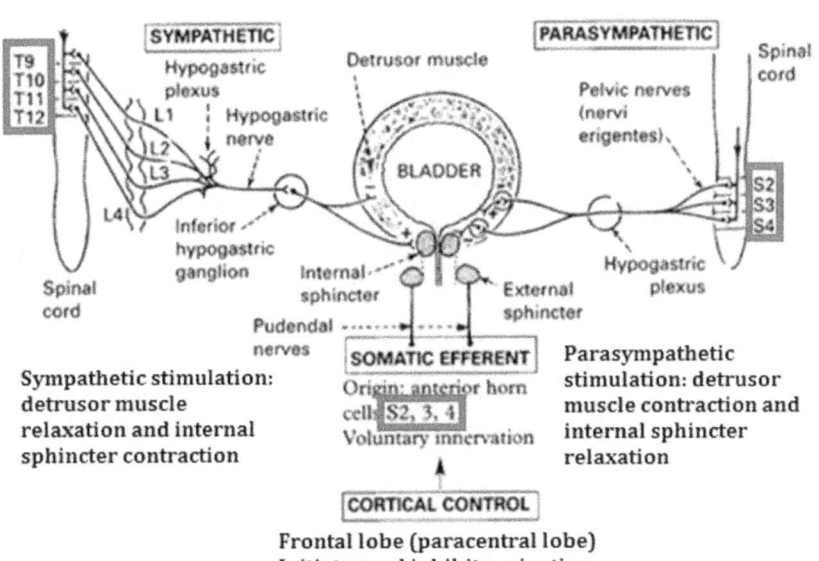

**A.4** Apart from radial pulse and tongue, you will want to do the following physical examination:

- Abdominal examination: look for bladder distention and masses (ovary, uterus, bowel content, kidneys, liver, and spleen)
- Perineal examination: look for prolapse
- Bimanual vaginal examination: look for prolapse

**A.5** Your management plan should basically include:

- Chinese herbal medicine and/or acupuncture-moxibustion treatments
- Urine diary
- Physiotherapist referral or self-educational materials for pelvic floor exercise (usually pelvic floor exercise takes three months to show effects)
- Development of coping strategy, for examples, avoidance of caffeine products, regular toileting, and wearing a pad

- Psychotherapy: cognitive behavioural therapy if you know how to do this, or simply taking therapy to relieve stress

---

# Revision Points

---

- Urinary system review questions: dysuria, discharge, change in frequency, change in colour, change in volume, hesitancy, urgency/leakage, and constipation. In male, you will also ask for strength of the stream and terminal dribbling.
- There are four common subtypes of urinary incontinence: urge incontinence, stress incontinence, mixed incontinence, and overflow incontinence.
- Nerve roots of the parasympathetic nervous system and somatic nervous system exit at the level of S2 to S4; and that of the sympathetic nervous system exit at the level of T9 to T12.
- Non-pharmacological treatment includes physiotherapy input, pelvic floor exercise, coping strategy, and psychotherapy.

# Type 1 diabetes in an 11-year-old girl

An 11-year-old girl presents with mother (who is an English teacher) to your Chinese medicine clinic for managements of his recently diagnosed type 1 diabetes at public general outpatient department. He has been having polydipsia and polyuria for three months. Her symptoms have resolved following administration of insulin. You have completed his Chinese medicine assessments and is currently developing his formula. At this time, her mother asks you the following questions:

Q.1 My daughter appears to be well. Why do we need treatments?

Q.2 I don't want my daughter to take insulin every day as you know, western medicine carries strong side-effects. Can we use Chinese herbal medicine to replace it?

Q.3 What should we do, if she is hypoglycaemic?

Q.4 Is having too much glucose in the body a bad thing?

Q.5 After using insulin for two months, my daughter does not require as much insulin as before. Is her diabetes going to be cured?

# Answers

**A.1** Having too much sugar in the blood for a short period of time does not cause any harm and the patient can be asymptomatic. However, if the blood sugar level remains high for a prolonged period of time, it can produce symptoms and complications. The classical symptoms of diabetes are polyuria, polydipsia, polyphagia, and a loss of weight. Despite children are more likely to present with classical signs, most do not. Adult seldom presents with classical signs.

A tight control of blood sugar level is important to prevent acute and chronic complications. Acute complications include diabetic ketoacidosis and hypoglycaemia (medical emergencies). Chronic complications include diabetic foot, cardiovascular disease (myocardial infarction), diabetic nephropathy, diabetic retinopathy, and diabetic neuropathy. In fact, poorly controlled diabetes is the main factor for chronic kidney disease, and cardiovascular disease is the leading cause of death in diabetic patients with poor control.

Type 1 diabetes is also associated with coeliac disease, Hashimoto's disease (hypothyroidism), polycystic ovarian syndrome, and gestational diabetes.

**A.2** You should advise the patient's mother that the side-effects of insulin are mainly hypoglycaemia and fat atrophy. And you should also mention the health consequence of not taking insulin, i.e. acute and chronic complications. You must not advise the patient to stop insulin, because this is not your expertise and this can kill the patient (this has happened before in Australia). While Chinese herbal medicines may be able to help with diabetes control, a sudden cessation of insulin is certainly not a wise option.

**A.3** In hypoglycaemic episode, the patient will experience symptoms including palpitation, sweating, anxiety, dizziness, and blackout, etc. The most common causes of hypoglycaemia are missed meals, alcohol use, too much exercise, and overdose of insulin. You should know about some key values:

- Coma occurs when blood sugar level (BSL) < 1.5 mmol/L
- Hypoglycaemia becomes dangerous when BSL < 3.0 mmol/L
- Hypoglycaemia occurs when BSL < 4.0 mmol/L

When the patient is hypoglycaemic yet conscious, patient or parent should:

- Finger prick BSL (optional)
- Rule of 15
    - 15 g of quick-acting carbohydrate (half can of Coca Cola)
    - Recheck finger prick BSL at 15 minutes (optional)
    - If the next meal is more than 15 minutes away, offer some long acting carbohydrate (sandwich)

- Recheck finger prick BSL at two to four hours (optional)
- Call ambulance if situation does not improve

**A.4** In diabetic ketoacidosis, the patient will be passing lots of urine (osmotic diuresis) to become dehydrated. The most common causes of this acute complication are urinary tract infection, myocardial infarction, pneumonia, and influenza. This is a highly dangerous condition and ambulance must be called immediately.

**A.5** Type 1 diabetes is not going to be cured. In fact, the patient not requiring as much insulin as before is likely to be due to honeymoon period. Honeymoon period usually occurs within the first year of diabetes, because at this time, the remaining pancreatic beta cells will continue to release as much insulin as possible. With disease progression, the remaining pancreatic beta cells died and the body can no longer produce insulin. This usually occur at 1 year. Therefore, you can expect the amount of insulin this girl requires will increase again at 1 year.

# Revision Points

- Classical symptoms of diabetes are polyuria, polydipsia, polyphagia, and a loss of weight. However, they are not common.
- Poor controlled diabetes lead to acute and chronic complications.
- Chinese medicine practitioners must not interfere with the usage of insulin and/or other medications that are not Chinese herbal medicines.
- Practitioners must not mistakenly think that using less amount of insulin during honeymoon period as a sign of cure or improvement.
- In hypoglycaemia, quick administration of quick-acting carbohydrate can be helpful. Remember the Rule of 15.
- In diabetic ketoacidosis, ambulance must be called immediately.

Your feedback is highly important to improve the content of this book. Please kindly send your feedback, opinions, or any mistakes that you have found in this book to my email address:

insectchia@yahoo.com.hk

Thank you.

# DISCLAIMER

All information published in this book represent the opinions of the author and do not reflect the views or policies of Chinese medicine societies in Australia and Hong Kong, or the publisher.

Some professionals in related disciplines may benefit from the informational content of this book. It is up to them to apply or reject it with professional jurisprudence.

The author assumes no responsibility for any injury and/or damage to persons or property arising from any use or execution of any methods, treatments, therapy, operations, instructions, ideas contained in this book.

The integration of Chinese medicine and biomedicine must begin by understanding each other, preferably using a common language. On top of that, mutual respect and appropriate use of knowledge, clinical skills, and interventions are of prime importance.

# ABOUT THE AUTHOR

Kwan Leung Chia, BChinMed (HK), is a practicing registered Chinese herbal medicine practitioner and acupuncturist in Australia and Hong Kong. He will soon finish his medical degree and start his career as medical intern/house officer.

His research interests include integrative medicine education, clinical practice model, medical acupuncture, clinical toxicology of herbal medicines, and emergency medicine. He is also an University Council Member of Flinders University and was Chairman of Chinese Medicine Society of Hong Kong University Students' Union.

www.ingramcontent.com/pod-product-compliance
Lightning Source LLC
Chambersburg PA
CBHW070333190526
45169CB00005B/1875